Jeffery Brown

# Soaring Above Negativity

# Contents



1.

2.

3.

4.

5.

6.

# 1

# Introduction

Overcoming negativity has a significant impact on one's mental health and well-being. Negativity, in the form of stress, anxiety, fear, and anger, can affect a person's thoughts, emotions, and behavior. When we are surrounded by negativity, it becomes easier to focus on the negative aspects of life and become more critical of ourselves and others. This type of negative thinking can lead to increased levels of stress and anxiety, which can, in turn, lead to physical and mental health problems.

On the other hand, overcoming negativity and adopting a positive outlook can have a profound impact on mental well-being. When you focus on the positive aspects of life, you become more resilient in the face of challenges, and you are more likely to feel satisfied with your life. Additionally, positive thinking can lead to improved relationships, increased creativity, and a greater sense of purpose. Therefore, overcoming negativity and adopting a positive outlook is an important aspects of mental health and well-being. Some strategies for overcoming negativity include mindfulness, gratitude, and seeking support from friends and family. Practicing positive self-talk, setting realistic goals, and engaging in activities that bring joy and fulfillment can also help to reduce negativity and improve mental health and well-being.

What is Negative Self-talk

Negative self-talk: This refers to the critical and demeaning thoughts we have about ourselves. Negative self-talk can include thoughts like, "I am not good enough," "I will never succeed," or "I am a failure." This type of negativity can be damaging to self-esteem and self-worth and can lead to feelings of depression and anxiety.

1. Pessimism: Pessimism is a general negative outlook on life and the future. Pessimistic people tend to see the glass as half empty, and they often focus on the negative aspects of situations rather than the positive. Pessimism can lead to feelings of hopelessness and a lack of motivation to try new things.

2. Cynicism: Cynicism is a skeptical and distrustful attitude towards others and the world. Cynics often view people and situations as being motivated by selfish or sinister intentions, and they can be quick to judge or criticize others. This negativity can lead to

feelings of anger and frustration and can make it difficult to form positive relationships with others.

It's important to recognize these forms of negativity and work to overcome them, as they can have a significant impact on mental health and well-being. By adopting a more positive outlook, setting realistic goals, and engaging in activities that bring joy and fulfillment, it is possible to reduce negativity and improve mental health and well-being.

It's important to note that change is possible and that you have the power to overcome negativity and improve your mental health and well-being. In this book, we will explore various steps that can help you achieve this goal, including:

1.  Understanding negativity: We will delve into the various forms that negativity can take, such as negative self-talk, pessimism, and cynicism, and examine the impact that these attitudes can have on mental health and well-being.

2.  Mindfulness and self-reflection: We will explore the concept of mindfulness and the importance of being present and aware of our thoughts, emotions, and physical sensations. We will also look at the role of self-reflection in overcoming negativity and developing a more positive outlook.

3.  Gratitude and positive thinking: We will discuss the benefits of adopting a grateful and positive mindset, and provide strategies for developing positive self-talk, setting realistic goals, and focusing on the positive aspects of life.

4.  Building resilience: We will examine the role that resilience plays in overcoming negativity and adapting to change, and provide tips and techniques for building resilience and coping with stress and adversity.

5.  Seeking support: We will explore the importance of seeking support from friends, family, and professionals, and provide guidance on how to build strong, supportive relationships.

By following these steps, you will learn how to overcome negativity, improve your mental health and well-being, and lead a more fulfilling life. So, let's get started on this journey toward positivity and growth.

# 2

# Chapter 1

Understanding Negativity

Negativity refers to a general attitude or state of mind characterized by an inclination to emphasize the bad or unpleasant aspects of things, people, or situations. This can manifest in various forms, including pessimism, cynicism, or critical thinking.

Negative emotions, on the other hand, are feelings that are unpleasant and are associated with negative events or thoughts. Some common negative emotions include:

- Anger
- Frustration
- Sadness
- Anxiety
- Despair
- Guilt
- Shame

- Envy

Common examples of negative behaviors include:

- Criticizing or blaming others
- Complaining and griping
- Engaging in negative self-talk
- Being argumentative or confrontational
- Avoiding or withdrawing from social interactions
- Holding grudges or harboring resentment
- Being overly suspicious or distrustful
- Being hostile, aggressive, or abusive towards others.

It's important to note that everyone experiences negative emotions and behaviors at times, and it is a normal part of the human experience. However, when negativity becomes chronic and excessive, it can have a negative impact on one's mental health and relationships.

Negativity can stem from a variety of causes, including childhood experiences, past traumas, and stress. Let's discuss each of these in more detail:

1. Childhood experiences: Childhood experiences can play a significant role in shaping a person's outlook on life and emotions. For example, growing up in an environment where there was little love, affection, or emotional support can lead to low self-esteem, a negative self-image, and a tendency to view the world as a harsh and unforgiving place. On the other hand,

if a child is raised in an environment of love, encouragement, and support, they are more likely to develop a positive outlook and an optimistic view of the world.

2. Past traumas: Traumatic events can leave deep emotional scars that affect a person for many years to come. For example, experiencing abuse, neglect, violence, or loss can lead to feelings of fear, anger, guilt, or shame. These feelings can shape a person's perception of the world, leading to negativity and a negative outlook.

3. Stress: Chronic stress can have a profound effect on a person's emotional well-being. When a person is constantly under stress, it can lead to feelings of anxiety, depression, and irritability. Over time, this can take a toll on a person's mental health, leading to a negative outlook on life.

It's important to note that while these are some of the root causes of negativity, they are by no means exhaustive. There may be other factors, such as biology, genetics, and personal circumstances, that can also contribute to a negative outlook. However, by understanding the root causes of negativity, people can work towards developing healthier and more positive coping mechanisms.

Negativity has a significant impact on the human body, both in terms of psychological and physiological responses. The brain is one of the primary targets of negative emotions, and prolonged exposure to stress and negativity can have a lasting impact on brain structure and function.

One of the key areas affected by negativity is the amygdala, which is responsible for regulating the body's stress response. When a person experiences negativity, the amygdala triggers the release of stress hormones, such as cortisol and adrenaline, which are designed to prepare the body for a fight-or-flight response. Prolonged exposure to elevated levels of cortisol can lead to damage to the hippocampus, which is involved in memory and learning, and can also lead to depression and anxiety.

Negativity can also impact other hormone systems in the body. For example, it can disrupt the delicate balance of hormones related to sleep, hunger, and metabolism, which can lead to insomnia, overeating, and weight gain.

Additionally, stress and negativity can weaken the immune system and make a person more susceptible to illness.

In conclusion, negativity has a significant impact on the human body, and its effects can be seen in the brain and various hormone systems. It is important to address and manage negativity in order to maintain physical and psychological well-being

Negativity can have a profound impact on relationships, work, and daily life. In relationships, negativity can cause tension, conflict, and mistrust, leading to breakdowns in communication, reduced intimacy, and even the end of the relationship. At work, negativity can create a hostile or toxic environment, leading to decreased productivity, increased stress levels, and high turnover rates. It can also damage relationships between coworkers and make it difficult to collaborate effectively. In daily life, negativity can be draining and can lead to decreased happiness and overall well-being. It can also impact physical health by increasing stress levels, which can lead to a range of health problems. Negativity can also impact one's perception of their own abilities and strengths. For example, negative self-talk can lead to decreased self-esteem and confidence and can make it difficult to approach tasks and situations with a positive mindset.

It's important to be aware of negativity and to take steps to counteract its effects. This can include setting healthy boundaries with negative people, practicing self-care and positive self-talk, and engaging in activities that bring joy and happiness into your life. Additionally, surrounding yourself with positive, supportive people can help to counteract negativity and promote a more positive outlook.

# 3

# Chapter 2

Mindfulness and Self-awareness

Mindfulness is a mental state achieved by focusing one's awareness on the present moment, while calmly acknowledging and accepting one's feelings, thoughts, and bodily sensations. It is a practice that originated from Buddhist meditation but has been widely adopted in the Western world for its numerous benefits, including reducing stress and improving overall well-being.

Regarding negativity, mindfulness can help overcome it in several ways. When we are mindful, we are better able to recognize negative thoughts and emotions as they arise, rather than getting caught up in them. This awareness provides us with the space to choose how we respond to these feelings, rather than being controlled by them. Instead of reactively responding to negative thoughts with more negativity, mindfulness helps us respond in a more positive and balanced way.

Additionally, mindfulness can also help us understand the root cause of our negative emotions. By taking a step back and observing our thoughts and feelings without judgment, we can gain insight into what is triggering these emotions and why. This understanding can help us address the underlying issue and reduce the frequency and intensity of negative emotions in the future.

In conclusion, mindfulness is a powerful tool that can help us overcome negativity by increasing our awareness of our thoughts and emotions, providing us with the space to respond in a positive and balanced way, and giving us the opportunity to understand and address the root cause of our negative feelings.

Mindfulness is a simple yet powerful technique for bringing greater awareness and presence to the present moment. Here are some tips and exercises to help you incorporate mindfulness into your daily life:

1. Start with deep breathing: Take a few deep breaths whenever you feel stressed or overwhelmed. Focus your attention on the sensation of breathing and try to let go of any distracting thoughts.

2. Practice mindfulness during routine activities: Try to be fully present and aware when you are brushing your teeth, taking a shower, or doing any other routine task. Pay attention to the sensation of the water on your skin, the taste of the toothpaste, and so on.

3. Use reminders: Put up post-it notes or set reminders on your phone to remind you to be mindful throughout the day.

4. Meditation: Regular meditation is one of the most effective ways to develop mindfulness. Try to set aside 10-15 minutes each day to sit quietly, focus on your breath, and let go of any thoughts or distractions.

5. Mindful eating: Pay close attention to the taste, texture, and sensations of your food as you eat. Avoid eating while doing other activities such as watching TV or using your phone.

6. Take a mindful walk: Take a walk in nature or in a quiet place and pay attention to your surroundings. Focus on the sensation of walking, the sounds around you, and the sights you see.

7. Be kind to yourself: Practice self-compassion and try to avoid criticizing yourself. Instead, focus on being kind and understanding towards yourself, just as you would towards a friend.

Remember, the key to developing mindfulness is to practice regularly, be patient with yourself, and stick with it even if it feels difficult at first. With time and practice, incorporating mindfulness into your daily life can bring greater peace, happiness, and well-being

Self-awareness is a crucial aspect of personal growth and development. It involves being conscious of one's thoughts, feelings, behaviors, and the impact they have on oneself and others. By having self-awareness, individuals are able to gain insight into their thoughts, emotions, and behaviors and how they influence their decisions and interactions.

One of the main benefits of self-awareness is that it allows individuals to recognize negative thought patterns and change them. Negative thought patterns are repetitive ways of thinking that lead to negative emotions, such as anxiety, depression, and low self-esteem. However, through self-awareness, individuals can identify when they are engaging in these negative thought patterns and take steps to change them.

For example, if someone has a negative thought pattern of constantly doubting their abilities, they may be able to recognize this thought pattern and challenge it by reframing their thoughts and focusing on their strengths. They may also try to practice mindfulness and become more aware of their thoughts as they occur, allowing them to catch negative thought patterns and change them before they become deeply ingrained.

In addition, self-awareness can also help individuals understand their motivations, values, and beliefs, which can help them make more informed decisions and set goals that are aligned with their personal values and desires.

In conclusion, self-awareness plays a vital role in recognizing and changing negative thought patterns. By gaining insight into one's thoughts, emotions, and behaviors, individuals can become more aware of negative thought patterns and take steps to change them. This can lead to improved mental health, better decision-making, and overall personal growth and development

.

Self-awareness and introspection are important skills that can help you understand your thoughts, feelings, motivations, and behaviors. Here are some exercises that you can try to develop these skills:

1.  Journaling: Writing down your thoughts and feelings on a regular basis can help you gain greater insight into your inner world. Try to write about a specific event or experience each day and reflect on your thoughts and feelings in that moment.

2. Meditation: Meditation is a powerful tool for developing self-awareness. Try practicing mindfulness meditation, where you focus on the present moment and observe your thoughts without judgment.

3. Self-reflection: Set aside time each day to reflect on your thoughts and emotions. Ask yourself questions like "What am I feeling right now?" and "What is causing me to feel this way?" This can help you understand the root causes of your emotions and thoughts.

4. Body scan: Lie down comfortably and close your eyes. Scan your body from head to toe, noticing any sensations or feelings you may have in each part. This can help you connect with your physical sensations and emotions.

5. Emotional intelligence assessment: There are various assessments available online that can help you better understand your emotional intelligence and provide insights into your strengths and weaknesses.

6. Gratitude practice: Take time to reflect on the things in your life that you are grateful for. This can help you cultivate a more positive outlook and increase self-awareness.

7. Seek feedback: Ask friends, family, or coworkers for their honest opinions and observations about you.

This can give you a different perspective on yourself and help you identify areas for improvement.

Remember, developing self-awareness and introspection is a lifelong journey, and it's important to be patient and persistent in your efforts.

# 4

# Chapter 3

Challenging Negative Thoughts

Negative thoughts can become self-fulfilling prophecies because the way we think about ourselves and the world around us can greatly impact our behavior and emotions. When we have negative thoughts, such as "I'm not good enough" or "I'll never succeed," we may act in ways that reinforce these beliefs. For example, if we believe we're not good enough, we may shy away from new challenges or not put as much effort into our work, which can then lead to poor performance and reinforce negative thoughts. Furthermore, our thoughts can also influence our emotions and well-being. If we consistently have negative thoughts, it can lead to feelings of sadness, anxiety, and low self-esteem, which can further impact our behavior and lead to a vicious cycle of negativity.

Moreover, these negative thoughts can become deeply ingrained in our thought patterns, making it difficult to challenge and change them. Over time, this can lead to a negative self-image and a limited outlook on life. Therefore, it's important to be aware of our negative thoughts and to try to challenge and replace them with positive, more constructive ones. This can help break the cycle of negativity and lead to a more fulfilling and optimistic outlook on life.

Here are some techniques for recognizing and challenging negative thoughts:

1.  Mindfulness: Becoming aware of negative thoughts as they arise and observing them without judgment can help you recognize patterns and gain insight into your thinking.
2.  Reframing: Reinterpret the situation or thought in a more positive or realistic light. For example, instead of thinking "I'm a failure" reframe it as "I made a mistake, but I can learn from it."
3.  Cognitive Restructuring: Identify and challenge negative thought patterns, such as overgeneralization or catastrophic thinking, and replace them with more balanced and realistic thoughts.

4. Behavioral Activation: Engage in activities that promote positive emotions and behaviors to counteract negative thoughts.
5. Gratitude Practice: Cultivate a daily practice of gratitude to shift focus towards positive experiences and emotions.
6. Cognitive-Behavioral Therapy: Seek professional help from a therapist trained in CBT, which is a form of psychotherapy that helps individuals identify and challenge negative thoughts and behaviors to improve emotional and mental well-being.

Here are some steps you can follow to replace negative thoughts with positive affirmations:

1. Identify negative thoughts: Pay attention to your inner voice and recognize the negative thoughts that pop up in your mind.
2. Challenge negative thoughts: Ask yourself if these negative thoughts are true or if there is evidence to support them.
3. Replace negative thoughts with positive affirmations: Once you have challenged negative thoughts, replace them with positive affirmations. These are positive

statements that reflect the way you want to think or feel.

4.  Repeat positive affirmations: Repeat you are positive affirmations to yourself daily, or as often as you need to.

5.  Believe in your positive affirmations: Believe in the positive affirmations you are telling yourself, and remind yourself that you are capable of achieving your goals and desires.

6.  Practice mindfulness: Be aware of your thoughts and try to catch any negative ones before they spiral out of control.

Remember that changing your thought patterns takes time and practice, so be patient with yourself and stay committed to the process

# 5

# Chapter 4

**B**uilding Resilience

esilience is the ability to adapt and bounce back from adversity, challenges, or stressful situations. It involves maintaining a positive attitude, being flexible, and finding ways to cope with difficulties. Resilience can help overcome negativity by providing a framework for responding to challenges in a constructive manner. Resilient individuals are better able to manage stress, maintain perspective, and stay focused on their goals. They also tend to be more optimistic, self-reliant, and persistent, which can help them overcome obstacles and setbacks. By cultivating resilience, individuals can build a foundation of emotional strength and resilience that enables them to cope with negative experiences and emerge stronger and more confident.

1. Develop a growth mindset: Approach challenges as opportunities for learning and growth.

2. Build a support network: Surround yourself with people who uplift and encourage you.
3. Practice gratitude: Focus on what you have rather than what you lack.
4. Engage in regular physical exercise: It can help reduce stress and improve mood.
5. Practice mindfulness: Mindfulness can help you become more aware of your thoughts and emotions, and manage them better.
6. Set realistic goals: Break big goals into smaller, more achievable steps.
7. Cultivate positive self-talk: Challenge negative self-talk and reframe it with positive affirmations.
8. Prioritize self-care: Get enough sleep, eat healthily, and make time for activities you enjoy.
9. Learn to adapt to change: Develop the flexibility to adapt to new situations and challenges.
10. Seek help when needed: It's okay to ask for help from friends, family, or a mental health professional when needed.

Self-care is important because it helps maintain our physical, mental, and emotional well-being, and allows us to better cope with stress and daily challenges. Here are some practical suggestions for prioritizing self-care:

1. Get enough sleep: Aim for 7-9 hours of sleep each night to feel rested and rejuvenated.
2. Eat a healthy diet: Consume a balanced diet with plenty of fruits, vegetables, lean proteins, and whole grains.
3. Exercise regularly: Engage in physical activity for at least 30 minutes a day to improve cardiovascular health, and mood, and reduce stress.
4. Practice mindfulness: Set aside time each day to meditate, practice deep breathing, or engage in other mindfulness techniques to reduce stress and promote relaxation.
5. Connect with others: Spend time with friends, and family, or engage in social activities to reduce feelings of isolation.
6. Engage in hobbies and activities that bring you joy: Engage in activities that help you unwind, relax and bring you happiness.
7. Take breaks: Take regular breaks throughout the day to recharge and avoid burnout.

Remember, self-care is an ongoing practice that requires intentional effort. Incorporating these habits into your daily routine can help improve your overall well-being and quality of life.

# 6

# Chapter 5

Surrounding Yourself with Positive figures

Surrounding yourself with positive people and experiences can have a significant impact on your mental and emotional well-being. Positive people can provide you with support, encouragement, and motivation, which can help you achieve your goals and overcome challenges. Positive experiences can bring you joy, happiness, and a sense of fulfillment, which can improve your overall quality of life. In contrast, negative people and experiences can drain your energy, increase stress and anxiety, and affect your mood and outlook. Therefore, choosing to surround yourself with positive influences can promote better mental and emotional health and lead to a more fulfilling and satisfying life.

1. Identify your needs and interests: Before building a support system, identify what kind of support you need and what interests you have. This can help you

find groups and organizations that align with your values and provide the type of support you require.

2.  Volunteer: Volunteering is a great way to meet like-minded people and contribute to a cause you believe in. It can also provide a sense of purpose and satisfaction.

3.  Seek therapy: Therapy can provide a safe and supportive environment to explore your thoughts and feelings. A therapist can also help you develop coping strategies and provide guidance on how to navigate difficult situations.

4.  Join social groups: Joining social groups, such as a book club, sports team, or hobby group, can provide an opportunity to meet new people with similar interests. This can help to build a sense of community and provide a support system for you.

5.  Maintain healthy relationships: Build and maintain healthy relationships with people who support you, listen to you, and offer encouragement. It's important to surround yourself with people who uplift and inspire you.

6.  Practice self-care: Taking care of yourself, physically and emotionally, is important in building a positive support system. This can include getting enough sleep, eating well, exercising regularly, and engaging in activities that make you happy.

To limit exposure to negativity, here are some strategies:

1.  Avoid toxic people: Identify people in your life who consistently bring negativity and try to limit your interactions with them. If possible, remove them from your life altogether.
2.  Limit social media use: Set boundaries on how much time you spend on social media each day. Consider using tools that track your usage or limit access during certain times.
3.  Curate your social media feed: Unfollow accounts that post negative or triggering content, and instead follow accounts that bring you joy and inspiration.
4.  Practice self-care: Engage in activities that bring you joy and help you recharge, such as exercise, meditation, or spending time with loved ones.
5.  Surround yourself with positivity: Seek out relationships with people who bring positive energy into your life, and participate in activities that promote positivity and personal growth.

Remember, it's important to prioritize your own well-being and mental health. Don't be afraid to set boundaries and remove yourself from negative environments in order to protect yourself.

# 7

# Conclusion

The power of your thoughts shapes your thoughts and influences your emotions and behavior, so it's important to cultivate a positive mindset. Practice gratitude. Focusing on what you're thankful for can shift your mindset and help you feel more positive.

Seek out relationships and environments that promote positivity and personal growth.

Building resilience and learning how to bounce back from setbacks and challenges, and use them as opportunities for growth.

Setting positive, realistic goals and taking action to achieve them. Positive thinking alone is not enough you need positive action to create a positive impact on the world.

Positive experiences can bring you joy, happiness, and a sense of fulfillment, which can improve your overall quality of life. In contrast, negative people and experiences can drain your energy, increase stress and anxiety, and affect your mood and outlook. Therefore, choosing to surround yourself with positive influences can promote better mental and emotional health and lead to a more fulfilling and satisfying life.

I wholeheartedly encourage you to embrace a positive outlook and continue to work towards creating a more fulfilling life for yourself. Surrounding yourself with positivity can help you build resilience, improve your mood, and enhance your overall well-being. Whether it's through cultivating positive relationships, seeking out enjoyable experiences, or simply focusing on the good in your life, taking steps to foster positivity can have a powerful impact on your happiness and success. So keep pushing forward with a positive attitude, and don't be afraid to seek out the support and resources you need to achieve your goals and create the life you truly want.